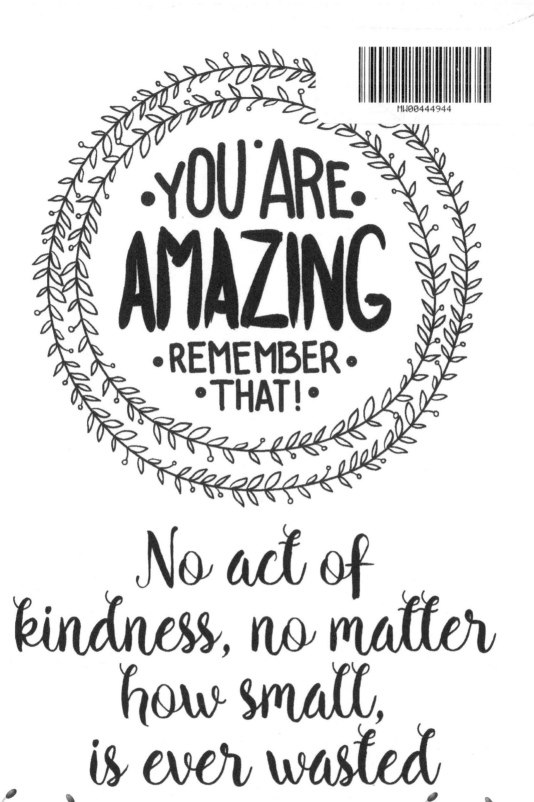

·YOU·ARE·
AMAZING
·REMEMBER·
·THAT!·

No act of
kindness, no matter
how small,
is ever wasted

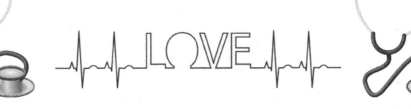

LOVE

# Nurse Life

○ MONDAY

PRIORITIES

○ TUESDAY

○ WEDNESDAY

TO DO

○ THURSDAY

○ FRIDAY

○ SATURDAY / SUNDAY

# MEALS / FOOD

# MISCELLANEOUS

| ME TIME - READ, WALK, RELAX, SPA, ETC | IMPORTANT STUFF | NOTES/REMINDERS | APPOINTMENTS | GROCERY SHOPPING | LIVE. LOVE. SLEEP. REPEAT. |
|---|---|---|---|---|---|
| | | | | | |
| | | | | | M |
| | | | | | T |
| | | | | | W |
| | | | | | T |
| | | | | | F |
| | | | | | S |
| | | | | | S |
| | | | | | |

## MONDAY

## TUESDAY

## WEDNESDAY

## THURSDAY

## FRIDAY

## SATURDAY-SUNDAY

# Nurse Life

○ MONDAY

PRIORITIES

○ TUESDAY

○ WEDNESDAY

TO DO

○ THURSDAY

○ FRIDAY

○ SATURDAY / SUNDAY

## MEALS / FOOD

## MISCELLANEOUS

## ME TIME - READ, WALK, RELAX, SPA, ETC

## IMPORTANT STUFF

## NOTES/REMINDERS

## APPOINTMENTS

## GROCERY SHOPPING

## LIVE. LOVE. SLEEP. REPEAT.

| | | | | | |
|---|---|---|---|---|---|
| | | | | | M |
| | | | | | T |
| | | | | | W |
| | | | | | T |
| | | | | | F |
| | | | | | S |
| | | | | | S |
| | | | | | |

## MONDAY

## TUESDAY

## WEDNESDAY

## THURSDAY

## FRIDAY

## SATURDAY-SUNDAY

# Nurse Life

○ MONDAY

PRIORITIES

○ TUESDAY

○ WEDNESDAY

TO DO

○ THURSDAY

○ FRIDAY

○ SATURDAY / SUNDAY

## MEALS / FOOD

## MISCELLANEOUS

| ME TIME - READ, WALK, RELAX, SPA, ETC | IMPORTANT STUFF | NOTES/REMINDERS | APPOINTMENTS | GROCERY SHOPPING | LIVE. LOVE. SLEEP. REPEAT. |
|---|---|---|---|---|---|
| | | | | | |
| | | | | | M |
| | | | | | T |
| | | | | | W |
| | | | | | T |
| | | | | | F |
| | | | | | S |
| | | | | | S |
| | | | | | |

## MONDAY

## TUESDAY

## WEDNESDAY

## THURSDAY

## FRIDAY

## SATURDAY-SUNDAY

# Nurse Life

○ MONDAY

PRIORITIES

○ TUESDAY

○ WEDNESDAY

TO DO

○ THURSDAY

○ FRIDAY

○ SATURDAY / SUNDAY

## MEALS / FOOD

## MISCELLANEOUS

| ME TIME - READ, WALK, RELAX, SPA, ETC | IMPORTANT STUFF | NOTES/REMINDERS | APPOINTMENTS | GROCERY SHOPPING | LIVE. LOVE. SLEEP REPEAT. | |
|---|---|---|---|---|---|---|
| | | | | | | M |
| | | | | | | T |
| | | | | | | W |
| | | | | | | T |
| | | | | | | F |
| | | | | | | S |
| | | | | | | S |
| | | | | | | |

## MONDAY

## TUESDAY

## WEDNESDAY

## THURSDAY

## FRIDAY

## SATURDAY-SUNDAY

# Nurse Life

○ MONDAY

PRIORITIES

○ TUESDAY

○ WEDNESDAY

TO DO

○ THURSDAY

○ FRIDAY

○ SATURDAY / SUNDAY

## MEALS / FOOD

## MISCELLANEOUS

| ME TIME - READ, WALK, RELAX, SPA, ETC | IMPORTANT STUFF | NOTES/REMINDERS | APPOINTMENTS | GROCERY SHOPPING | LIVE. LOVE. SLEEP. REPEAT. |
|---|---|---|---|---|---|
| | | | | | |
| | | | | | M |
| | | | | | T |
| | | | | | W |
| | | | | | T |
| | | | | | F |
| | | | | | S |
| | | | | | S |
| | | | | | |

## MONDAY

## TUESDAY

## WEDNESDAY

## THURSDAY

## FRIDAY

## SATURDAY-SUNDAY

## MEALS / FOOD

## MISCELLANEOUS

| ME TIME - READ, WALK, RELAX, SPA, ETC | IMPORTANT STUFF | NOTES/REMINDERS | APPOINTMENTS | GROCERY SHOPPING | LIVE. LOVE. SLEEP. REPEAT. |
|---|---|---|---|---|---|
| | | | | | |
| | | | | | M |
| | | | | | T |
| | | | | | W |
| | | | | | T |
| | | | | | F |
| | | | | | S |
| | | | | | S |
| | | | | | |

## MONDAY

## TUESDAY

## WEDNESDAY

## THURSDAY

## FRIDAY

## SATURDAY-SUNDAY

# Nurse Life

○ MONDAY

PRIORITIES

○ TUESDAY

○ WEDNESDAY

TO DO

○ THURSDAY

○ FRIDAY

○ SATURDAY / SUNDAY

# MEALS / FOOD

# MISCELLANEOUS

| ME TIME - READ, WALK, RELAX, SPA, ETC | IMPORTANT STUFF | NOTES/REMINDERS | APPOINTMENTS | GROCERY SHOPPING | LIVE. LOVE. SLEEP. REPEAT. |
|---|---|---|---|---|---|
| | | | | | |
| | | | | | M |
| | | | | | T |
| | | | | | W |
| | | | | | T |
| | | | | | F |
| | | | | | S |
| | | | | | S |
| | | | | | |

# MONDAY

# TUESDAY

# WEDNESDAY

# THURSDAY

# FRIDAY

# SATURDAY-SUNDAY

# Nurse Life

○ MONDAY

PRIORITIES

○ TUESDAY

○ WEDNESDAY

TO DO

○ THURSDAY

○ FRIDAY

○ SATURDAY / SUNDAY

## MEALS / FOOD

## MISCELLANEOUS

| ME TIME - READ, WALK, RELAX, SPA, ETC | IMPORTANT STUFF | NOTES/REMINDERS | APPOINTMENTS | GROCERY SHOPPING | LIVE. LOVE. SLEEP. REPEAT. |
|---|---|---|---|---|---|
| | | | | | |
| | | | | | M |
| | | | | | T |
| | | | | | W |
| | | | | | T |
| | | | | | F |
| | | | | | S |
| | | | | | S |
| | | | | | |

## MONDAY

## TUESDAY

## WEDNESDAY

## THURSDAY

## FRIDAY

## SATURDAY-SUNDAY

# Nurse Life

○ MONDAY

PRIORITIES

_____

○ TUESDAY

_____

○ WEDNESDAY

TO DO

_____

○ THURSDAY

_____

○ FRIDAY

_____

○ SATURDAY / SUNDAY

_____

## MEALS / FOOD

## MISCELLANEOUS

| ME TIME - READ, WALK, RELAX, SPA, ETC | IMPORTANT STUFF | NOTES/REMINDERS | APPOINTMENTS | GROCERY SHOPPING | LIVE. LOVE. SLEEP. REPEAT. |
|---|---|---|---|---|---|
| | | | | | M |
| | | | | | T |
| | | | | | W |
| | | | | | T |
| | | | | | F |
| | | | | | S |
| | | | | | S |
| | | | | | |

## MONDAY

## TUESDAY

## WEDNESDAY

## THURSDAY

## FRIDAY

## SATURDAY-SUNDAY

# Nurse Life

○ MONDAY

PRIORITIES

○ TUESDAY

○ WEDNESDAY

TO DO

○ THURSDAY

○ FRIDAY

○ SATURDAY / SUNDAY

## MEALS / FOOD

## MISCELLANEOUS

## ME TIME - READ, WALK, RELAX, SPA, ETC

## IMPORTANT STUFF

## NOTES/REMINDERS

## APPOINTMENTS

## GROCERY SHOPPING

## LIVE. LOVE. SLEEP. REPEAT.

| | | | | | | |
|---|---|---|---|---|---|---|
| | | | | | | M |
| | | | | | | T |
| | | | | | | W |
| | | | | | | T |
| | | | | | | F |
| | | | | | | S |
| | | | | | | S |
| | | | | | | |

## MONDAY

## TUESDAY

## WEDNESDAY

## THURSDAY

## FRIDAY

## SATURDAY-SUNDAY

# Nurse Life

○ MONDAY

PRIORITIES

_____

_____

○ TUESDAY

_____

_____

_____

_____

○ WEDNESDAY

TO DO

_____

○ THURSDAY

_____

_____

_____

_____

○ FRIDAY

_____

_____

_____

_____

○ SATURDAY / SUNDAY

_____

_____

_____

## MEALS / FOOD

## MISCELLANEOUS

| ME TIME - READ, WALK, RELAX, SPA, ETC | IMPORTANT STUFF | NOTES/REMINDERS | APPOINTMENTS | GROCERY SHOPPING | LIVE. LOVE. SLEEP. REPEAT. |
|---|---|---|---|---|---|
| | | | | | |
| | | | | | M |
| | | | | | T |
| | | | | | W |
| | | | | | T |
| | | | | | F |
| | | | | | S |
| | | | | | S |
| | | | | | |
| | | | | | |

## MONDAY

## TUESDAY

## WEDNESDAY

## THURSDAY

## FRIDAY

## SATURDAY-SUNDAY

# Nurse Life

○ MONDAY

PRIORITIES

_____

○ TUESDAY

_____

○ WEDNESDAY

TO DO

○ THURSDAY

_____

○ FRIDAY

_____

○ SATURDAY / SUNDAY

_____

## MEALS / FOOD

## MISCELLANEOUS

| ME TIME - READ, WALK, RELAX, SPA, ETC | IMPORTANT STUFF | NOTES/REMINDERS | APPOINTMENTS | GROCERY SHOPPING | LIVE. LOVE. SLEEP. REPEAT. |
|---|---|---|---|---|---|
| | | | | | |
| | | | | | M |
| | | | | | T |
| | | | | | W |
| | | | | | T |
| | | | | | F |
| | | | | | S |
| | | | | | S |
| | | | | | |

## MONDAY

## TUESDAY

## WEDNESDAY

## THURSDAY

## FRIDAY

## SATURDAY-SUNDAY

# Nurse Life

○ MONDAY

PRIORITIES

○ TUESDAY

○ WEDNESDAY

TO DO

○ THURSDAY

○ FRIDAY

○ SATURDAY / SUNDAY

## MEALS / FOOD

## MISCELLANEOUS

| ME TIME - READ, WALK, RELAX, SPA, ETC | IMPORTANT STUFF | NOTES/REMINDERS | APPOINTMENTS | GROCERY SHOPPING | LIVE. LOVE. SLEEP. REPEAT. |
|---|---|---|---|---|---|
| | | | | | |
| | | | | | M |
| | | | | | T |
| | | | | | W |
| | | | | | T |
| | | | | | F |
| | | | | | S |
| | | | | | S |
| | | | | | |

## MONDAY

## TUESDAY

## WEDNESDAY

## THURSDAY

## FRIDAY

## SATURDAY-SUNDAY

# Nurse Life

○ MONDAY

○ TUESDAY

○ WEDNESDAY

○ THURSDAY

○ FRIDAY

○ SATURDAY / SUNDAY

PRIORITIES

TO DO

## MEALS / FOOD

## MISCELLANEOUS

| ME TIME - READ, WALK, RELAX, SPA, ETC | IMPORTANT STUFF | NOTES/REMINDERS | APPOINTMENTS | GROCERY SHOPPING | LIVE. LOVE. SLEEP. REPEAT. |
|---|---|---|---|---|---|
| | | | | | |
| | | | | | M |
| | | | | | T |
| | | | | | W |
| | | | | | T |
| | | | | | F |
| | | | | | S |
| | | | | | S |
| | | | | | |

## MONDAY

## TUESDAY

## WEDNESDAY

## THURSDAY

## FRIDAY

## SATURDAY-SUNDAY

# Nurse Life

○ MONDAY

PRIORITIES

○ TUESDAY

○ WEDNESDAY

TO DO

○ THURSDAY

○ FRIDAY

○ SATURDAY / SUNDAY

# MEALS / FOOD

# MISCELLANEOUS

| ME TIME - READ, WALK, RELAX, SPA, ETC | IMPORTANT STUFF | NOTES/REMINDERS | APPOINTMENTS | GROCERY SHOPPING | LIVE. LOVE. SLEEP. REPEAT. |
|---|---|---|---|---|---|
| | | | | | |
| | | | | | |
| | | | | | M |
| | | | | | T |
| | | | | | W |
| | | | | | T |
| | | | | | F |
| | | | | | S |
| | | | | | S |
| | | | | | |

## MONDAY

## TUESDAY

## WEDNESDAY

## THURSDAY

## FRIDAY

## SATURDAY-SUNDAY

# *Nurse Life*

○ MONDAY

PRIORITIES

○ TUESDAY

○ WEDNESDAY

TO DO

○ THURSDAY

○ FRIDAY

○ SATURDAY / SUNDAY

## MEALS / FOOD

## MISCELLANEOUS

| ME TIME - READ, WALK, RELAX, SPA, ETC | IMPORTANT STUFF | NOTES/REMINDERS | APPOINTMENTS | GROCERY SHOPPING | LIVE. LOVE. SLEEP. REPEAT. |
|---|---|---|---|---|---|
| | | | | | |
| | | | | | M |
| | | | | | T |
| | | | | | W |
| | | | | | T |
| | | | | | F |
| | | | | | S |
| | | | | | S |
| | | | | | |

## MONDAY

## TUESDAY

## WEDNESDAY

## THURSDAY

## FRIDAY

## SATURDAY-SUNDAY

# Nurse Life

○ MONDAY

PRIORITIES

○ TUESDAY

○ WEDNESDAY

TO DO

○ THURSDAY

○ FRIDAY

○ SATURDAY / SUNDAY

## MEALS / FOOD

## MISCELLANEOUS

| ME TIME - READ, WALK, RELAX, SPA, ETC | IMPORTANT STUFF | NOTES/REMINDERS | APPOINTMENTS | GROCERY SHOPPING | LIVE. LOVE. SLEEP. REPEAT. |
|---|---|---|---|---|---|
| | | | | | |
| | | | | | M |
| | | | | | T |
| | | | | | W |
| | | | | | T |
| | | | | | F |
| | | | | | S |
| | | | | | S |
| | | | | | |

## MONDAY

## TUESDAY

## WEDNESDAY

## THURSDAY

## FRIDAY

## SATURDAY-SUNDAY

# Nurse Life

○ MONDAY

PRIORITIES

_____

○ TUESDAY

_____

○ WEDNESDAY

TO DO

_____

○ THURSDAY

_____

○ FRIDAY

_____

○ SATURDAY / SUNDAY

_____

## MEALS / FOOD

## MISCELLANEOUS

## ME TIME - READ, WALK, RELAX, SPA, ETC

## IMPORTANT STUFF

## NOTES/REMINDERS

## APPOINTMENTS

## GROCERY SHOPPING

## LIVE. LOVE. SLEEP. REPEAT.

| | | | | | | |
|---|---|---|---|---|---|---|
| | | | | | | M |
| | | | | | | T |
| | | | | | | W |
| | | | | | | T |
| | | | | | | F |
| | | | | | | S |
| | | | | | | S |

## MONDAY

## TUESDAY

## WEDNESDAY

## THURSDAY

## FRIDAY

## SATURDAY-SUNDAY

## MEALS / FOOD

## MISCELLANEOUS

| ME TIME - READ, WALK, RELAX, SPA, ETC | IMPORTANT STUFF | NOTES/REMINDERS | APPOINTMENTS | GROCERY SHOPPING | LIVE. LOVE. SLEEP. REPEAT. |
|---|---|---|---|---|---|
| | | | | | |
| | | | | | M |
| | | | | | T |
| | | | | | W |
| | | | | | T |
| | | | | | F |
| | | | | | S |
| | | | | | S |
| | | | | | |

## MONDAY

## TUESDAY

## WEDNESDAY

## THURSDAY

## FRIDAY

## SATURDAY-SUNDAY

# Nurse Life

○ MONDAY

PRIORITIES

_____

_____

○ TUESDAY

_____

_____

_____

_____

_____

○ WEDNESDAY

TO DO

_____

○ THURSDAY

_____

_____

_____

_____

○ FRIDAY

_____

_____

_____

○ SATURDAY / SUNDAY

_____

_____

_____

## MEALS / FOOD

## MISCELLANEOUS

| ME TIME - READ, WALK, RELAX, SPA, ETC | IMPORTANT STUFF | NOTES/REMINDERS | APPOINTMENTS | GROCERY SHOPPING | LIVE. LOVE. SLEEP. REPEAT. |
|---|---|---|---|---|---|
| | | | | | |
| | | | | | M |
| | | | | | T |
| | | | | | W |
| | | | | | T |
| | | | | | F |
| | | | | | S |
| | | | | | S |
| | | | | | |

## MONDAY

## TUESDAY

## WEDNESDAY

## THURSDAY

## FRIDAY

## SATURDAY-SUNDAY

# Nurse Life

○ MONDAY

PRIORITIES

_____
_____

○ TUESDAY

_____
_____
_____
_____

○ WEDNESDAY

TO DO

_____
_____

○ THURSDAY

_____
_____
_____
_____

○ FRIDAY

_____
_____
_____
_____

○ SATURDAY / SUNDAY

_____
_____
_____

## MEALS / FOOD

## MISCELLANEOUS

| ME TIME - READ, WALK, RELAX, SPA, ETC | IMPORTANT STUFF | NOTES/REMINDERS | APPOINTMENTS | GROCERY SHOPPING | LIVE. LOVE. SLEEP. REPEAT. |
|---|---|---|---|---|---|
| | | | | | |
| | | | | | M |
| | | | | | T |
| | | | | | W |
| | | | | | T |
| | | | | | F |
| | | | | | S |
| | | | | | S |
| | | | | | |

## MONDAY

## TUESDAY

## WEDNESDAY

## THURSDAY

## FRIDAY

## SATURDAY-SUNDAY

# Nurse Life

○ MONDAY

○ TUESDAY

○ WEDNESDAY

TO DO

○ THURSDAY

○ FRIDAY

○ SATURDAY / SUNDAY

## MEALS / FOOD

## MISCELLANEOUS

## ME TIME - READ, WALK, RELAX, SPA, ETC

## IMPORTANT STUFF

## NOTES/REMINDERS

## APPOINTMENTS

## GROCERY SHOPPING

## LIVE. LOVE. SLEEP. REPEAT.

| | | | | | |
|---|---|---|---|---|---|
| | | | | | M |
| | | | | | T |
| | | | | | W |
| | | | | | T |
| | | | | | F |
| | | | | | S |
| | | | | | S |
| | | | | | |

## MONDAY

## TUESDAY

## WEDNESDAY

## THURSDAY

## FRIDAY

## SATURDAY-SUNDAY

# Nurse Life

○ MONDAY

PRIORITIES

○ TUESDAY

○ WEDNESDAY

TO DO

○ THURSDAY

○ FRIDAY

○ SATURDAY / SUNDAY

## MEALS / FOOD

## MISCELLANEOUS

| ME TIME - READ, WALK, RELAX, SPA, ETC | IMPORTANT STUFF | NOTES/REMINDERS | APPOINTMENTS | GROCERY SHOPPING | LIVE. LOVE. SLEEP. REPEAT. |
|---|---|---|---|---|---|
| | | | | | |
| | | | | | M |
| | | | | | T |
| | | | | | W |
| | | | | | T |
| | | | | | F |
| | | | | | S |
| | | | | | S |
| | | | | | |

## MONDAY

## TUESDAY

## WEDNESDAY

## THURSDAY

## FRIDAY

## SATURDAY-SUNDAY

# Nurse Life

○ MONDAY

PRIORITIES

_____
_____
_____
_____
_____

○ TUESDAY

_____
_____
_____
_____

○ WEDNESDAY

TO DO

_____
_____
_____

○ THURSDAY

_____
_____
_____
_____

○ FRIDAY

_____
_____
_____
_____

○ SATURDAY / SUNDAY

_____
_____
_____
_____

## MEALS / FOOD

## MISCELLANEOUS

| ME TIME - READ, WALK, RELAX, SPA, ETC | IMPORTANT STUFF | NOTES/REMINDERS | APPOINTMENTS | GROCERY SHOPPING | LIVE. LOVE. SLEEP. REPEAT. | |
|---|---|---|---|---|---|---|
| | | | | | | M |
| | | | | | | T |
| | | | | | | W |
| | | | | | | T |
| | | | | | | F |
| | | | | | | S |
| | | | | | | S |
| | | | | | | |

## MONDAY

## TUESDAY

## WEDNESDAY

## THURSDAY

## FRIDAY

## SATURDAY-SUNDAY

# Nurse Life

○ MONDAY

PRIORITIES

○ TUESDAY

○ WEDNESDAY

TO DO

○ THURSDAY

○ FRIDAY

○ SATURDAY / SUNDAY

## MEALS / FOOD

## MISCELLANEOUS

| ME TIME – READ, WALK, RELAX, SPA, ETC | IMPORTANT STUFF | NOTES/REMINDERS | APPOINTMENTS | GROCERY SHOPPING | LIVE. LOVE. SLEEP. REPEAT. |
|---|---|---|---|---|---|
| | | | | | M |
| | | | | | T |
| | | | | | W |
| | | | | | T |
| | | | | | F |
| | | | | | S |
| | | | | | S |
| | | | | | |

## MONDAY

## TUESDAY

## WEDNESDAY

## THURSDAY

## FRIDAY

## SATURDAY-SUNDAY

# Nurse Life

○ MONDAY

PRIORITIES

○ TUESDAY

○ WEDNESDAY

TO DO

○ THURSDAY

○ FRIDAY

○ SATURDAY / SUNDAY

## MEALS / FOOD

## MISCELLANEOUS

ME TIME - READ, WALK, RELAX, SPA, ETC

IMPORTANT STUFF

NOTES/REMINDERS

APPOINTMENTS

GROCERY SHOPPING

LIVE. LOVE. SLEEP. REPEAT.

M
T
W
T
F
S
S

## MONDAY

## TUESDAY

## WEDNESDAY

## THURSDAY

## FRIDAY

## SATURDAY-SUNDAY

# *Nurse Life*

○ MONDAY

PRIORITIES
_____
_____
_____
_____
○ TUESDAY
_____
_____
_____
_____

○ WEDNESDAY

TO DO
_____
_____
○ THURSDAY
_____
_____
_____
_____
_____
○ FRIDAY
_____
_____
_____
_____
_____
○ SATURDAY / SUNDAY
_____
_____
_____
_____

## MEALS / FOOD

## MISCELLANEOUS

| ME TIME - READ, WALK, RELAX, SPA, ETC | IMPORTANT STUFF | NOTES/REMINDERS | APPOINTMENTS | GROCERY SHOPPING | LIVE. LOVE. SLEEP. REPEAT. |
|---|---|---|---|---|---|
| | | | | | |
| | | | | | M |
| | | | | | T |
| | | | | | W |
| | | | | | T |
| | | | | | F |
| | | | | | S |
| | | | | | S |
| | | | | | |

## MONDAY

## TUESDAY

## WEDNESDAY

## THURSDAY

## FRIDAY

## SATURDAY-SUNDAY

# Nurse Life

○ MONDAY

PRIORITIES

_____

○ TUESDAY

○ WEDNESDAY

TO DO

○ THURSDAY

○ FRIDAY

○ SATURDAY / SUNDAY

Made in the USA
Middletown, DE
20 May 2019